MW01166070

Disclaimer

This book contains content generated by us. The content in this book is provided for general information only. It is not intended to amount to advice on which you should rely. In particular, this information is not a substitute for professional medical care by a qualified doctor or other healthcare professional. If you are not a healthcare professional then you should ALWAYS check with your doctor if you have any concerns about your condition or treatment and before taking, or refraining from, any action on the basis of the content on our book. If you are a healthcare professional then this information (including any professional reference material) is intended to support, not replace, your own knowledge, experience and judgement.

Copyright

services. If advice is necessary, legal or professional, a practiced individual in the profession should be ordered.

Table of Contents

Vitamin D

Chapter 1

Definition of a Nutrient

„I believe that the greatest gift you can give your family and the world is a healthy you."

Joyce Meyer

We all talk a lot about nutrition and eating "nutrient rich" food. But, what exactly is a nutrient? How is it so essential to our body? And what are the functions it performs in the body? Simply put, a nutrient is said to be a component in the food that living beings need for survival and growth purposes. Nutrients can be classified in two categories:

Macronutrients: These are the heavy hitters which provide the body with the energy to carry out the various metabolic functions. The body requires these nutrients to be consumed in large quantities.

Micronutrients: Though not major, these components provide the body with the cofactors which aid in the actual functioning of the metabolic processes. The requirement of these nutrients is less and should be consumed in small quantities. Both, macronutrients and micronutrients, are readily available in the environment. They have a lot of functions to perform in the body and they provide the body with energy, help in regulating the bodily processes and aid in building new tissues and repairing the old and damaged ones. Plants and animals have different ways to intake the nutrients from the environment. Plants absorb the required nutrients from the soil through their roots and the leaves absorb the nutrients from the atmosphere. Animals have a digestive system that breaks down the foods consumed and extract the macronutrients and micronutrients from it. The macronutrients are then used for energy purposes and micronutrients are used to aid in and carry out various metabolic activities in the body.

Organic Nutrients: Proteins, carbohydrates, vitamins and fats

Inorganic Nutrients: Water, oxygen and dietary minerals.

So this is the basic definition of a nutrient. Each and every food item we consume has one or more nutrients present in it, some more than the other. To keep our body healthy it is absolutely essential that we try and consume a variety of nutrient rich foods so that our body receives all the nutrients required to carry out metabolic functions. Say if you only consume junk food like French fries, all your body is getting is carbohydrates, fats and sodium. So your body gets energy from the food, but as junk food is not rich in the micronutrients, your body cannot perform metabolic functions and that energy is going waste. In recent times, experts realized that by meeting the requirements of both, micronutrients and macronutrients, it does not necessarily mean that a person will lead a healthy life. This point was proved by the increasing amount of different diseases in the western countries. The ratio of the people suffering from heart diseases, cancer, and obesity is high in such countries.

The reason for this is the increasing amount of junk food in people's diets and the reducing amount of physical activity. Good, balanced meals should always be accompanied by some sort of physical activity to ensure that you remain healthy and disease free for life.

Summary of Chapter 1

Nutrients can be classified in two categories:

- Micronutrients
- Macronutrients.

The macronutrients are then used for energy purposes and micronutrients are used to aid in and carry out various metabolic activities in the body.

There are also:

- Organic Nutrients
- Inorganic nutrients (water and minerals)

Chapter 2

The Important Nutrients

„Health is not valued till sickness comes."

Thomas F.

All nutrients are important, but some are more important than the others. Most people manage to consume an appropriate amount of nutrients by chance, but they are not aware of the exact ratio of the nutrients that are necessary for growth. On a daily basis, each individual uses or loses some amount of nutrients while performing different activities. In case there is a shortage of a particular nutrient in the body, the tissues present in the body use the stored nutrients to fulfill the requirement. But, if proper nutrients are not consumed and stored, there will be a shortage of nutrients, leading to a deficiency.

A mentioned before, some nutrients have a more important role in our body. Here are some of the nutrients which play a very important role in the body:

1. Proteins

The word is derived from a Greek word, which means, holding the first place. Proteins are the root cause of the existence of a living organism. Proteins are made from amino acids, which are also known as the building blocks of the body. Protein is mainly found in, milk, butter, bread, cereals, and meat. People, who are vegetarian, consume protein from legumes, fruits, vegetables and other dairy products. Vegans mainly derive their protein from soy based products.

2. Fats

The main property of fat is that they are not soluble in water, but they are soluble in an organic substance, known as acetone. The texture of fat is greasy, and non-volatile. Fats help in performing both, structural and metabolic functions in the body.

Health experts describe fats in two forms, i.e. visible and invisible. Visible fats are those, which we can see with our naked eyes, these include olive oil, butter, cheese or sunflower spread and fat in meat pieces. While invisible fats include products like, junk food, pastries, egg yolk, etc., where you physically cannot see the fat content of the product.

3. Carbohydrates

Carbohydrates are the set of substances that are usually found in both, plants and animals. Though carbohydrates are not an essential nutrient, they are considered important as they are one of the major sources of energy for the body. Carbohydrates are present in a variety of foods like vegetables, cereals, pulses, dairy products, etc. Usually carbohydrates are found in processed foods. (d) Vitamins Vitamins are said to be organic compounds which play a vital role in a lot of the bodily metabolic processes. Vitamins can either be fat soluble or water soluble, depending on their chemical build up. There are 14 known vitamins and some of the rich sources of these vitamins are lean meats, dairy products, green leafy vegetables, yellow and orange fruits and vegetables.

Summary of Chapter 2

Most people manage to consume an appropriate amount of nutrients by chance, but they are not aware of the exact ratio of the nutrients that are necessary for growth.

Nutrient have more important role in our body. Here are some of the nutrients which play a very important role in the body:

1. Proteins
2. Fats
3. Carbohydrates

Chaptep 3

Vitamin D

„When wealth is lost, nothing is lost; when health is lost, something is lost; when character is lost, all is lost."

B. Graham

Early researches based on Vitamin D started from the disease rickets. Rickets is a bone disease, which is usually seen in infants and in early childhood. In the year 1919, Sir Edward Mellanby proved that the disease is caused due to the lack of the nutrition and he also proved that the disease could be cured with the help of the sunlight. Over the span of the next few years various scientists, with the help of different experiments and studies, researched the benefits of UV rays on children suffering from rickets and proved that the nutrient gained from sunlight had a very large impact on children who suffered from rickets. Vitamin D is defined to be a group of secosteroids which are fat soluble in nature. This group of secosteroids aids the intestine in absorbing magnesium, iron, calcium, zinc and phosphate.

As far as humans are concerned, cholecalciferol (vitamin D3) and ergocalciferol (vitamin D2) are extremely important for growth and developmental purposes. The body cannot produce these

Vitamin D compounds internally and it is required that we try and include vitamin D in our diet and expose ourselves to the sun to synthesize vitamin D in our body.

Types Of Vitamin D

There are several types of vitamin D based on their chemical composition. The two major types of vitamin D are ergocalciferol (vitamin D2) and cholecalciferol (vitamin D3).

Just plain vitamin D without any subscript refers to either ergocalciferol or cholecalciferol or even both. Vitamin D3 and Vitamin D2 together are known as calciferol. In 1931, the chemical composition of vitamin D2 was characterized and the chemical structure of vitamin D3 was proven in the year 1935 after researching the effect of 7 dehydrocholestrol on UV rays.

The different types of vitamin D are chemically known as secosteroids. Secosteroids are said to be the steroids with one broken steroid bond in their ring. The vitamin is divided into the following types based on their chemical composition

1. Vitamin DI

2. Vitamin D.

3. Vitamin D3

4. Vitamin D4

5. Vitamin D5

Summary of Chapter 3

Vitamin D is defined to be a group of secosteroids which are fat soluble in nature. This group of secosteroids aids the intestine in absorbing magnesium, iron, calcium, zinc and phosphate.

The two major types of vitamin D are ergocalciferol (vitamin D2) and cholecalciferol (vitamin D3).

The vitamin is divided into the following types based on their chemical composition

1. Vitamin DI

2. Vitamin D.

3. Vitamin D3

4. Vitamin D4

5. Vitamin D5

Chapter 4

Factors Affecting The Production Of Vitamin D

„The excitement of vitamins, nutrition and metabolism permeated the environment."

Paul D. Boyer

Numerous biological factors affect the production or synthesis of Vitamin D3 in the body. All these factors, primarily include, ageing, style of clothing, exposure to the sunlight, excessive use of the sunscreen lotions, various types of pollutions and the different seasons. Among all of the reasons, degree of pigmentation and ageing is the most important one.

1. Pigmentation in Skin

Lesser amounts of solar radiation and skin pigmentation are the two issues that affect the production of Vitamin D3. This is mainly due to the presence of melanin that fights against the 7 dehydrocholesterol, and prevents the absorption of the ultra-violate rays that are essential for vitamin D3 synthesis in the body.

2. Aging

As you grow older, you skin gets thinner. This entire process begins after you have crossed the age of twenty. The level of the seven-dehydrocholesterol keeps on increasing with your growing age, but the production of vitamin D3 does not increase due to the thinning skin. A young adult can make about three times more vitamin D than his or her elders. As the time passes, the thickness of your skin keeps on decreasing, resulting less production of the vitamin.

3. Sunscreen

Usage It is important to apply sunscreen lotion when you move out in the sun, as it protects your skin from getting sunburned, and from diseases like skin cancer. The main issue with sunscreens is that they stop the good radiations that help in the production of the vitamin D3 in your body.

4. Seasons

Seasons also affect the production of vitamin D in your body. In cold areas the seven dehydrocholesterol is in effect for a short period. As the summers are short the seven dehydrocholesterol is active in those few days. But in such a short time it is difficult for the body to create vitamin D3 in large amounts. That is the reason why most people in such countries prefer spending the summer days lounging in the sun and getting tanned.

Summary of Chapter 4

There are 4 major factors that can affect the production of Vitamin D. These factors are:

- Sunscreen
- Aging
- Pigmentation in Skin
- Seasons

Chapter 5

Hidden Benefits Of Vitamin D

„To keep the body in good health is a duty... otherwise we shall not be able to keep our mind strong and clear."

Buddha

Vitamin D is essential in the human body for various activities. One of the most important activities, which require vitamin D, is bone growth. Vitamin D helps calcium to get absorbed in the body of any living organism and as we all know calcium is essential for bone development in the body. Apart from that, the vitamin is also helpful for the growth and development of the heart muscles, fat tissues and brain cells. Vitamin D governs the different cell development, and cell growth activities in the body and that is why it is an essential nutrient for our body. In addition to this, it also helps in the metabolic control and the immune functions taking place in the body. In the past few years vitamin D has gained popularity. The vitamin led all the experts to have an endless debate.

Some studies claim that the vitamin D, individually, does not have any outcome specifically, but when it gets associated with other processes, it is very beneficial. Whereas, some other studies claim that the blood vessels containing the vitamin have high percentage of toxins that result in some serious cardiovascular problems in the body. This can cause to the premature death of an individual.

Vitamin D for Weight Loss

„It is health that is real wealth and not pieces of gold and silver."

Gandhi

Scientists believe that the vitamin D has too many things to offer human beings. It has the hidden answers to some of the most discussed and controversial studies. Earlier, it was assumed that the vitamin could help cure cancer, cardiac problems and even aid in weight loss. There were no proofs that the vitamin can actually help in weight loss, until a group of scientist of Fred Hutchinson Cancer Research Center, who were studying a few overweight women suffering from the deficiency of vitamin D. They discovered that the women lost some weight over a span of 12 months. These women were taking a continuous, and a fixed amount of vitamin D supplements. Apart from that, they were following a daily exercise routine. The scientists also observed that the women, who were on the brim of being deficient, became even slimmer. The weight loss on both the types of groups was very normal. When these women were compared with the women, who had followed a proper diet, the results were quite similar. In the end, the experts concluded their research with positivity that vitamin D could help to treat health problems like obesity.

The Relation Of Calcium And Vitamin D

In order to live a healthy life, it is very important to have strong and solid bones. Calcium is one of the minerals that is very essential for the survival of a living organism. Together, vitamin D and calcium, play the most important circle that makes a living organism live for many years. Calcium is one of the elements that keeps the bones healthy. This is not it; it also helps in the clotting of our blood, and sends messages to the nerves, resulting in the contraction of the muscles. Looking at the ratio of the calcium in the body of the human beings, about 90 percent of it is in the bones as well as in the teeth. It is also present in the skin, hair, nails, urine, and even in sweat. Therefore, every day we lose some amount of calcium from our body and hence, it needs to be replenished on a daily basis.

1. Calcium

In The Body Bones contain a special compartment for the fluids, which is separated from other sections. The compartment of bone mainly comprises a space filled with the fluid, in between the thin linings of the cells and the matrix of the bone. Therefore, the fluid is in the direct contact with the bones.

The ratio of the calcium in the bone fluid is normally about one third than in the other fluids, for example, in extracellular fluid. There are small lining cells on the outer side of the bone and the fluid. These small cells have some open channels that permit the entry of calcium in the fluid of the bones. The movement of the fluid towards the upward direction involves a transportation process that can pump it through the lining of the cells.

2. Bones and vitamin D

It has been proved that vitamin D is required for the normal and smooth development of the bones. It also helps in the mineralization process, which leads to the remodeling of bones. Researches have also suggested the role of vitamin D in the development of the bone is major as it helps in passing calcium form one stage to another. It further helps calcium to get absorbed in the sections of the bones. This entire procedure is supported by the increased absorption level of minerals in the intestines.

Convenient Sources Of Vitamin D

Vitamin D is not very commonly found in foods. Perhaps this is why the skin gains the vitamin lot of the vitamin from sunlight. When it comes to the food items, liver oils of fish, and fatty fishes, such as tuna, pilchards, and herring are some of the examples of the rich sources of the vitamin D. Other than, fishes, it is also found in the liver of the mammals and dairy products, like milk based beverages, but the quantity of the vitamin is too low. Food products like vegetables, fruits, and cereals carry zero percent of vitamin D. This is why most vegans and vegetarians are at a high risk of getting a vitamin D deficiency and are advised to spend a lot of time out in the sun or, in extreme cases, take vitamin D supplements.

Summary of Chapter 5

1. Vitamin D is essential in the human body for various activities. One of the most important activities, which require vitamin D, is bone growth. Vitamin D helps calcium to get absorbed in the body of any living organism and as we all know calcium is essential for bone development in the body.

2. Vitamin D governs the different cell development, and cell growth activities in the body.

3. The experts concluded their research with positivity that vitamin D could help to treat health problems like obesity.

4. Vitamin D is not very commonly found in foods.

5. Other than, fishes, it is also found in the liver of the mammals and dairy products, like milk based beverages, but the quantity of the vitamin is too low.

6. Most vegans and vegetarians are at a high risk of getting a vitamin D

Chapter 6

Vitamin D Deficiency

As explained before, the main factors that affect the formation of Vitamin D in the body include dark skin tone, lack of sunlight, breastfeeding and that too without any supplements. In the case of the vitamin D deficiency, the production of the calcium binding protein decreases. Therefore, when the calcium presented in the body travels without the presence of this binding protein, it passes through without being absorbed. With the deficiency of vitamin D, the adolescents may not live a healthy life, and they will suffer from massive amounts of calcium deficiency. This increase in the deficiency can lead the child to suffer from various other chronic diseases.

1. Osteomalacia

When you are too young, your body needs a fixed amount of Vitamin D. And as the age increases, the requirement of the vitamin remains constant, but the skin gets too thin, and with prolonged ageing the skin is not able to synthesize it. This leads them to have horrible pain all night long and at times swelling. With the deficiency of Vitamin D, the bones get too soft and fragile, and in some cases, deformed. (1) Rickets Rickets is the most popular and most common disease in children. The percentage of the children suffering from the disease is higher in the developing and under developed countries. Tibet, Mongolia and Netherlands are a few examples of the countries which have a lot of children that are suffering from rickets. Even in the developed countries like United States of America, there are numerous cases of the disease reported. A major part of children who suffer from it, have a dark complexion. The number of baby girls suffering from rickets is higher than that of the boys. In order to prevent the spread of this disease, the government of America provides several injections or medicines to provide the vitamin to their body and help prevent and cure the disease. In the disease, the bones of the patient get really weak. This is because the bones do not get the required amount of calcium to maintain its strength. In order to support their entire body, these kids bend a little and walk, spoiling their posture for life.

2. Osteoporosis

When the body of a human being does not get enough quantity of vitamin D, from their food or from the sun, they have weak bones. This is because of vitamin D is mainly responsible for the absorption of calcium in the body and its transportation in the body. It also helps the bones to soak the calcium in order to gain some mass and strength. Osteoporosis literally means "porous bones" in Greek. In this disease the density and the mass of the bones decrease, leading to an increased risk of getting a fracture. The bone mineral density (BMD) decreases and results in increased instances of falling and bone breakage in people suffering from it. The disease is most commonly seen in women, and women patients outnumber the male patients in a ratio.

3. Elders

As we have already discussed above, that with the growing age, the production of vitamin D, keeps on decreasing. When an individual reaches his or her old age, their different body parts do not work properly. In other words, their internal organs like, kidney, liver, and skin create very less amount of vitamin D, which is not enough for the proper working of the entire body. As a result, most of the times, elderly spend a major part of their time in their homes. This stops their body from absorbing some amount of Vitamin D from the sun. Even if they step out of their homes, they wear layers of

Vitamin D

clothes, in which, again, gets impossible for the UV rays to get in touch with their skin. In the end, all such things, affects their bones, making them even weaker and softer for their body structure.

Infertility

„The management of fertility is one of the most important functions of adulthood."

G. Greer

4. Female

The ratio of infertility varies from percent to percent in 30-40% of cases one partner suffers from infertility. The rest of the ratio, i.e. 20-40% of cases are not aware about the real cause, while there are some couples in which, both of the partners are infertile. After many researches, and experiments, experts were able to prove that change with seasons and climatic conditions can also affect the sperm quality and the ovulation ratio as well. In various studies, women were provided with versions of vitamin D3, along with some amount of calcium, and phosphorus. After some time, women who were not able to conceive earlier, were now able to have a successful mating, and now they have a healthy litter. With the above studies, scientists found out that Vitamin D alone does not cause infertility. However, it is associated with calcium and phosphorus. In addition to this, they also found that climatic temperature and conditions also play a vital role.

5. Male

In the above-mentioned case, we have already discussed about the infertility ratio in one of the partners. Various studies earlier have proved that, vitamin D has affected the male reproductive system in male animals. In humans, vitamin D is the agent that exerts the mechanism and various related functions of the male reproductive system and the entire process. It affects the agents like, cholesterol efflux, protein, increases the calcium levels, and allows a spontaneous and independent move, leading to the survival of the sperm. Studies proved that men with Vitamin D deficiency had lower rates of the sperm movement than that of the men with normal rate of Vitamin D.

After many years of research and studies, scientists proved that the decreasing ratio of testosterone's in men is caused due to many factors, and low ratio of vitamin D is one of all the reasons. However, its role in infertility is more than in females.

6. Insulin Secretion

Dihydroxyvitamin D3 is said to be the agent that helps in the secretion of the insulin. Studies proved that the change in the ratio, of vitamin D, that carries a protein in the pancreas and in other parts of the body, might affect the entire process of the secretion of insulin.

Other Effects On The Body

1. Cardiovascular problems

For the past few years, doctors and experts have been associating the deficiency of Vitamin D with the cardiovascular system. These studies got an approval from the different medical institutes, when the cardiac patients were observed with kidney related diseases. The death ratio of the patients who are suffering from such renal diseases is about 20 percent higher than that of the normal patients. As the functioning of the kidney of an individual starts deteriorating, its level of calcitriol also declines, resulting in the improper production and functioning of other agents presented in it. This leaves a direct effect on the various nutrients and organs of the body. Vitamin D is the most important molecule for the better functioning of the heart, as it keeps various cardiovascular diseases at a distance. If there is a deficiency of vitamin D in the body, the defenses of the heart go down, giving way for a lot of diseases to creep in.

2. Different Infections

Vitamin D plays a vital role in helping your body to fight with the immune system against the various viruses. Most of the time, these viruses cause common colds and other such minor diseases. A study at Massachusetts General Hospital, Boston proved that the people with low level of vitamin D are more prone to catching a cold.

3. Cancer

In the last 20 years, dermatologists have proved that among all the factors that causes cancer, the major on is vitamin D, and the deficiency of the secretion of insulin. Above we have explained how vitamin D affects the secretion of insulin; therefore, at the end less vitamin D is one of the main culprits of causing cancer. Let us begin by explaining how cancer grows in the body of an individual. It starts with the increasing percentage of the cells. Normally, when a certain amount of cells are dying, a fixed amount of cells take birth to replace those dying cells. In the death of the old cells, vitamin D plays a vital role. Whereas for the birth of the new cells insulin plays a key role. Without Vitamin D, the death of the cells will be affected. On the other hand, insulin will keep on producing new cells. This will result in the excessive amount of the cells in the body. These cells later take a bunch form or form knots; the prominent symptom of cancer. Another reason, which causes deficiency of vitamin D, is Insulin Resistance Syndrome (IRS). This is caused due to obesity. Physicians have proved that obesity plays an important role in the formation of cancerous cells in the body.

4. Type 2 Diabetes

Vitamin D plays an important role in the proper functioning of the immune system. Deficiency of Vitamin D can imbalance the functioning of the immune system. As a result, your immune system goes into autoimmune mode and kills all the cells producing insulin in the pancreas. Once the production of insulin is stopped in the body, evolution of Type 1 diabetes set in. Studies have found that most of the diabetic patients suffer from the deficiency of vitamin D. Doctors dealing with the diabetic patients prefer to check the level of vitamin D before they begin with their normal diabetic treatment. This test helps them in getting a clear view of the main reason behind the person getting type 1 diabetes. These days even teenagers suffer from diabetes. As a treatment for diabetes, most of the time, doctors prefer giving them some supplements that will help them to regain their insulin level. These supplements usually are vitamin D supplements, in the hope that the surge of vitamin D in the body will help balance the immunity system and stop the autoimmune activity against the pancreas. If they are not provided with the supplements on time, they will have to follow the normal diabetic treatment for their entire life.

5. Blood Pressure

In medical terms, high blood pressure is known as hypertension. In the past few years, the percentage of the high blood pressure has increased at a fast rate. In a study, researchers discovered that the cases of hypertension were more in the places that are far from the equator. This simply meant that farther you stay from heat or direct sunlight, the higher are the chances of you suffering from high blood pressure.

High blood pressure is caused due to the following three pointers:

1. Over acceleration of the RAAS, also known as `Renin angiotensin Aldosterone System'.
2. The resistance of insulin.
3. The mechanism of neurons, from the mind to the body.

As explained before, resistance to insulin is an indirect effect of lack of vitamin D in the body.

Summary of Chapter 6

Vitamin D deficiency can cause:

1. 2. Osteoporosis
2. Osteomalacia
3. Elders
4. Infertility
5. Insulin Secretion

Vitamin D definiciency can cause the following effect on the body:

1. Cardiovascular problems
2. Different Infections
3. Cancer
4. Type 2 Diabetes
5. Blood Pressure

Chapter 7

Excessive Consumption Of Vitamin D

A vitamin is an essential molecule in the body of a living organism. We all know about the role vitamin D plays in the absorption of calcium in the body and the transport of calcium to the various body parts. More than that, it also helps it to get absorbed in the bones. However, excessive amounts of vitamin D can be extremely dangerous for all. Until now, we have learned on how vitamin D helps a living organism to live a healthy life. We also talked about how the deficiency vitamin D can lead to numerous amounts of diseases which may be fatal in the long run.

Toxicity of Vitamin D

Vitamin D is extremely helpful and is very important for the various functions in the body. But, its excess amount can bring some major troubles for you. The fat-soluble vitamin is can have some toxic effect if it is consumed in large amount. The amount of vitamin, which is made within our skin, and which is consumed with the food products is sufficient for our body to function properly, and that is the safest ratio for the consumption of the Vitamin D. At times, people who are deficient in the vitamin D take different types of supplements, in order to create a balanced amount of Vitamin D in their body. But, they should keep one thing in mind that the supplement should not be given to children. The body of a child is capable enough to create its own vitamin in the natural way. Even the adults are prescribed to use the vitamin supplement in a fixed ratio and for a fixed period.

Excess of Vitamin D can raise the concentration of calcium in the blood. Blood with the excessive amount of calcium can destroy all the soft tissues, which further leads to the creation of the stones, which later get collected in the kidney, in an attempt for secretion.

Conclusion

As you can see, vitamin D is extremely important for the proper functioning of the body. The lack if this vitamin has many side effects — some of them fatal. It is essential that you try and include as many sources of vitamin D in your diet as you can and spend some time out in the sun so that your body can synthesize the vitamin from the UV rays. Get regular blood tests done to ensure that you are consuming the correct amount of vitamin D and the vitamin D levels in your body are at a perfect level; not too low nor too high. Do not self diagnose and start with supplements without consulting with your general physician or doctor. Before doing anything always take the advice of your physician; you never know, you may end up doing more harm than good. Also, a word of caution. Do not be out in the sun for too long, lest you get sunburnt or increase the risk getting skin cancer!

Follow the guidelines written in this eBook to ensure that you live a healthy, disease free life. Thank you for downloading this eBook and we hope that you found the content of this eBook informative and it helps you lead a healthy life.

Huge Thank You and Words of Gratitude!

First and foremost, Thank You for downloading this book. At the end of the day I'm **extremely** grateful for **every** download and **every** purchase. It really makes me smile and motivates me. I wish that every person would put their best forward for the human race. I wish you unlimited mental strength and discipline to achieve your goals and dreams. **Together** we can make the difference.

If you found the information useful I would be extremely grateful if you could write a short Amazon review. It really does make the difference and I personally read every review and take notes. I want to improve my books, so that I can provide more value to other people. I know that my future books will give you the best experience possible.

Download this book in Mp3 for FREE

I want to give you a little bonus for your purchase.

Please visit this link: http://eepurl.com/bsBSAL

Made in the USA
Las Vegas, NV
19 February 2025

18409513R00026